THE DMSO REVOLUTION HANDBOOK GUIDE.

A BREAKTHROUGH IN MODERN HEALTHCARE.

…for the treatment of Spinal Cord Injuries, Carpal Tuned Syndrome (CTS), Diabetes, Cancerous Growth, Arthritis, Facial Acne, Stroke, Burns, Shingles & Herpes, Ear & Eye Infections, Nerve Pain, Brain Injuries & Retardation, Cirrhosis of The Liver, Fibromyalagia, Fungus, Hair-Scalp, Headaches, Interstitial Cystitis, Lupus, Stroke, Spinal Cord, Tooth & Gum Diseases.

By

JANE K. JEREMY

<u>**DISCLAIMER.**</u>

This book's content is written and published strictly for educational and informational purpose(s) only. It is not intended to be a medical prescriptional treatment, except under the strict supervision of a certified healthcare specialist.

This book is not intended for diagnosing any challenging health condition, and it is not a potential alternative for a medical practitioner. Always consult the services of a medical expert for medical counsel before engaging in the prescriptions documented on this book.

Table of Contents.

CHAPTER 1. 8

DMSO: A BRIEF HISTORY...8

IS DMSO TOXIC?..16

CHAPTER 2...18

CLINICAL BENEFITS OF HEALING OF DMSO....18

HOW TO APPLY DMSO TO THE BODY.............18

▶ TOPICAL APPLICATION:...............................19

DMSO APPLICATION IN FACIAL TREATMENT.
....20

▶ ORAL APPLICATION:.......................................22

CHAPTER 3...25

CHEMICAL REACTION OF DMSO WITH WATER.
....25

HOW TO EXTRACT DMSO FROM WATER
SOLUBLE...25

HOW DMSO AFFECTS PREGNANT WOMEN
AND NURSING MOTHERS..26

✥ ALOE VERA AND DMSO. 27

CRYOPROTECTANT DIMETHYL SULPHOXIDE...29

DMSO FOR THE TREATMENT OF FACIAL ACNE. 31

HOW DMSO RELATES TO CELL-BIOLOGY AND THE VITRO-FERTILIZATION PROCESS.33

AMYLOIDOSIS. 35

CHAPTER 4...37

ALZHEMER'S, ARTHRITIS, HERPES, SHINGLES, ATHLETIC INHURIES, NERVE PAIN, BRIAN AND DEMENTIA DISEASES. 37

ALZHEMER'S 37

ARTHRITIS...38

HERPES AND SHINGLES. 40

NERVE PAIN. 42

ATHLETIC INJURIES.......................................43

BRAIN INJURIES. 45

Industrial or vehicular accidents. 45

⧗ Falls. 45

⧗ Trauma. 45

CHAPTER 5 48

BURNS, CANCER, CARPAL TUNNEL SYNDROME, AND CIRRHOSIS OF THE LIVER ...48

↳ CANCER AND CANCEROUS GROWTH. 49

↳ CARPAL TUNNEL SYNDROME. 51

↳ CIRRHOSIS OF THE LIVER. 54

DIABETES, DIGESTIVE, EAR & EYE INFECTIONS PROBLEMS. 55

↳ DIABETES. 55

↳ DIGESTIVE PROBLEMS 58

↳ EAR INFECTIONS 59

↳ EYE DISEASES 61

CHAPTER 7 63

FIBROMYALAGIA, FUNGUS, HAIR-SCALP, AND HEADACHES. 63

↳ DMSO AS AN ANTI-FUNGAE AGENT. 65

✹   HAIR AND SCALP PROBLEMS. 66

✹   HEADACHES. 68

CHAPTER 8 70

INTERSTITIAL CYSTITIS, LUPUS, STROKE, SPINAL CORD, TOOTH & GUM DISEASES. 70

✹   INTERSTITIAL CYSTITIS. 70

✹   LUPUS. 72

✹   STROKE, AND SPINAL CORD INJURIES...74

✹   TOOTH AND GUM DISEASE. 76

CHAPTER 9 81

STORAGE & INDUSTRIAL USE OF DMSO. 81

✹   DMSO As A Cleaning Agent & Processing Agent: 81

✹   DMSO As A Radiation Protective Agent. 82

HOW TO STORE DMSO? 83

CHAPTER 1.

DMSO: A BRIEF HISTORY.

The Dimethyl sulfoxide was actually first processed as a solvent suitable for industrial use, by a Russian Chemist/scientist known as Alexander Saytzeff. While on a research routine, he noticed that the substance had a garlic-like odor, it was odorless, oily while touched, and left an aftertaste similar to clams or oysters.

Experimentally, it was found out that dimethyl sulfoxide (DMSO) was an excellent solvent, that is used as a degreaser, paint thinner, and as an antifreeze. It is used also as an excellent industrial solvent with regards to antibiotics, plant hormones, herbicides for the control of weeds, as well as fungicides.

In the twentieth century, scientists examined DMSO use as an anti-inflammatory agent, as they discovered that when it was spilled on the hands during experiments, the individual scientists experienced some kind of garlic-like taste on their tongues/taste buds.

After World War II, being fascinated by the skin-to-taste effect, researchers began to make inquiries as to how the liquid could easily permeate the skin.

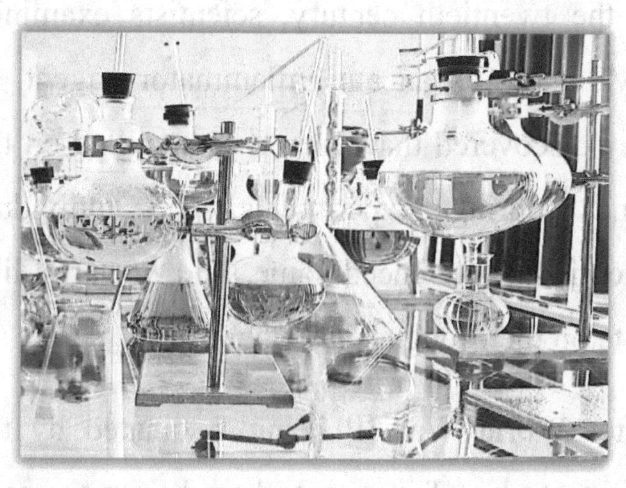

In the year 1965, the Food & Drugs Administration (FDA) suspended the proposed clinical trials by enumerating the potential safety concerns, which is a result of the adverse effects of the eye lenses and visual that is associated with the use of the substance. At this point, DMSO was seen as a very toxic solvent compared to thalidomide.

A couple of years later, after some experiments on animals, DMSO was in use again by man. From that time onwards, DMSO has been in use for some selected medical applications in human medicine, including being used as an organ preservative, for treating cryopreservation of stem cells, interstitial cystitis, treatment of musculoskeletal and dermatological diseases, treatment of increased intracranial pressure, etc.

In the year 1978, the FDA approved the use of DMSO in a 50:50 ratio mixture with water as an effective treatment for the symptoms of interstitial cystitis. And from that time till now, a whole lot of people have received this treatment.

<u>GETTING TO KNOW DMSO: THE WONDER DRUG.</u>

The Dimethyl sulfoxide, also known as DMSO, is generally a naturally occurring chemical substance, and it is one of the components of the world's complex sulphuric cycle.

It is noticeable in natural water, soil, and some selected foods like milk, tea, tomatoes, and crops to be present at low concentrations <0.05ppm to 3.7 ppm. Generally, the metabolism of DMSO in soil by microorganisms results in forming sulfur and dimethyl sulfide.

DMSO has been approved for use in other pharmaceutical formulations in the United States of America and other countries, around the World. Also, in the year 1998, the FDA endorsed the recommendation of the expert working group of the International Conference on Harmonization relative to the residual solvents in pharmaceuticals.

Therefore, DMSO was placed in the safest category; **_Class-III_** solvents, with low toxic potential. This class of solvent includes the solvents known for minimal health hazards, at levels normally accepted in Pharmaceuticals. Solvents in Class-III may be regarded as less toxic and of lower risk to human health.

The Dimethyl Sulfoxide (DMSO) is a commercially produced organic polar aprotic solvent with an amphipathic nature that is known to be best at dissolving poorly soluble polar and non-polar molecules.

13

For emphasis, it is a clear and odorless liquid. It is gotten cheaply from the pine trees as a by-product of the paper-making industry and is now a prescribed medicine and dietary supplement, remarkably versatile in therapy.

DMSO can be administered by mouth, applied to the skin (dermally or topically), or injected intravenously into the veins.

Just like any other chemical compound, DMSO has its own unique physical properties. These include the following;

1. It has a relatively high boiling point and an organic liquid that is miscible in water. Boiling points 190°C/375°F, and a melting point of 65.2°F.

2. It is odorless and exhibits low toxicity, with a pressure of vapor 0.44mmHg at a temperature of 67°F.

3. DMSO is a highly polar, dipolar aprotic solvent, with a Density of 1.105 at 69°F.

4. Dimethyl Sulfoxide is a highly solvent soluble in chloroform, acetone, ethanol, benzene, and ether.

5. It is highly hygroscopic. Molecular Weight of 76.24 g/mol.

IS DMSO TOXIC?

In a research, sixty (60) prisoners in California volunteered to have DMSO in an 80% gel applied to their skin at one-gram-per-kilogram for a period of fourteen (14) days, and they were reported to have no toxic effects. A second group of forty (40) prisoners allowed themselves to be coated with DMSO and had no toxicological result.

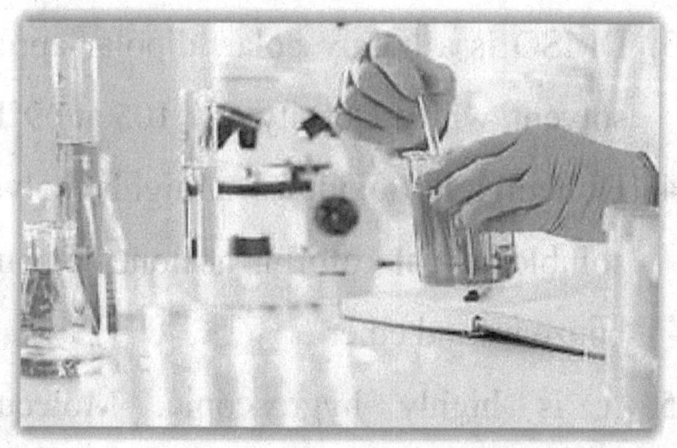

These persons' eyes were examined with the help of a slit lamp, and an ophthalmoscope. They were examined both for lens refraction and visual fields. These individuals also went through urine, liver, blood, and other analyses.

There were so many more studies on the DMSO's toxicology for about 3-months after the experiment, and researchers finally came to the conclusion that the DMSO drug is safe and good for human consumption.

CHAPTER 2.

CLINICAL BENEFITS OF HEALING OF DMSO.

One of the chemical benefits of DMSO is that it reacts with heavy metals like nickel, cadmium, lead, aluminum, and mercury, by detoxifying them (through sweating, urination, and also defecation).

HOW TO APPLY DMSO TO THE BODY.

There are three practiced ways/methods of applying DMSO to the human or animal's body. These methods include; Intravenous, Oral, and Topical.

▶ <u>INTRAVENOUS APPLICATION:</u>

Another way/method of administering the dimethyl sulfoxide is through the use of injection shots (intravenous method).

There are some ailments that cannot be treated effectively with the oral or topical methods of application, but only through intravenous means, for faster relief.

Ailments such as chronic inflammatory bladder disease, and others.

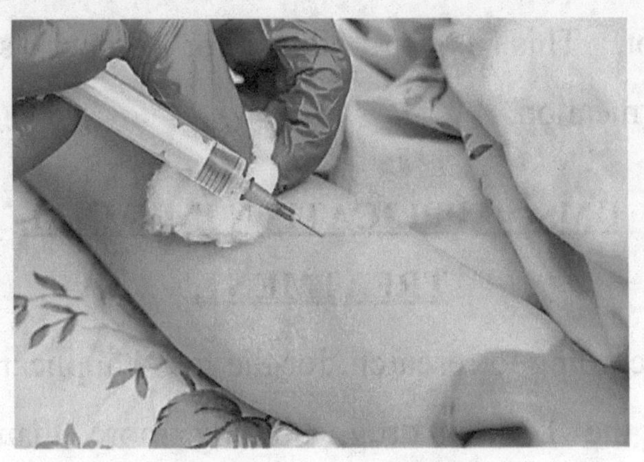

▶ __TOPICAL APPLICATION:__

Here, DMSO is generally administered in liquid or jelly form. DMSO helps in no small way to stimulate the quick recovery of the affected body area from burns, pains, injuries, and wounds.

You can also apply dimethyl sulfoxide in the treatment of headaches, bodily inflammations, and other ailments. Gently apply the liquid or gel substance to the surface/or the spot of impact and leave for about 30 minutes on the spot. This is to allow for proper skin permeation.

DMSO APPLICATION IN FACIAL TREATMENT.

According to research, for the facial application of the DMSO drug, nothing more than a concentration of 20% should be applied to the facial and neck regions of the body.

Beginning a DMSO treatment with a lower concentration/dosage of this drug before progressing to a much higher concentration is strongly advised, regardless of the method of administration.

To achieve a perfect mix for the treatment discussed, gently mix a 10ml of water to a 65% DMSO concentration, and gently rub it on your skin (at the target area). Rub it luxuriously for about 5 times daily for the next two days.

Applying a DMSO conc. that is above 80 to 90% without adequate mixing compliment to your face, neck, and tender regions, could result in a gradual wrinkling, and irritations of that part of the body.

▶ <u>ORAL APPLICATION:</u>

This is usually done with the help of a teaspoon. The amount of dosage administered in the oral administration of DMSO is normally measured in ml.

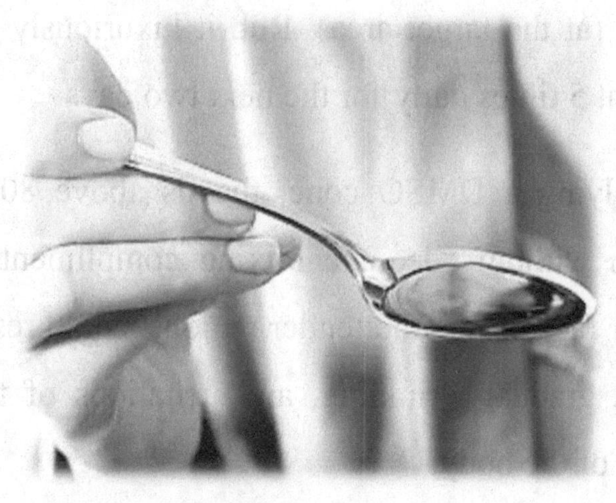

From scientific studies, the allowable dosage of the DMSO drug in an oral administration is a maximum of two teaspoons in a day, and its concentration should not be more than 5%. And because of its nature, being that it has a very strong and pungent smell, it is best mixed with some juice, to help mask the smell and its garlic-like taste.

THE NEXT TURN.

CHAPTER 3.

CHEMICAL REACTION OF DMSO WITH WATER.

The dimethyl sulfoxide is a chemical solvent that is highly soluble in water. Chemically, DMSO has six atoms of hydrogen in its chemical formation and water has two atoms in its chemical formation. These atomic properties enable them to magnetize each other and quicken the solubility between water and DMSO.

HOW TO EXTRACT DMSO FROM WATER SOLUBLE.

There are basically three ways of extracting DMSO from a water-soluble. These procedures include:

To concentrate the already diluted water and DMSO mixture to about 70%, then remove the non-volatile physical and chemical impurities through the process of evaporation. Lastly, to recover the pure DMSO substance, through the fractional distillation process(es) of the solution.

HOW DMSO AFFECTS PREGNANT WOMEN AND NURSING MOTHERS.

Expectant and nursing mothers as well as their infant child should seldomly be administered with DMSO, except otherwise prescribed by a qualified and trusted medical doctor.

In fact, it is recommended that its application should be thoroughly avoided during pregnancy. Alternative medications should be used in these cases. This is because researchers have come to the realization that administering DMSO to pregnant women has an adverse effect on the unborn child because DMSO permeates the skin down to the blood streams which supplies nutrients to the unborn child. The same also applies to breast-feeding women, as they can transmit DMSO through the breast milk to their infant/suckling children.

✍ **ALOE VERA AND DMSO.**

Aloe vera is a plant with many health benefits. It is used both in the beauty and cosmetic industry as well as in the field of medicine.

Aloe vera when squeezed, the fluid can be used to mix creams for better enhancement of the skin. When Aloe-vera fluid of 50% conc. is mixed with DMSO of 50% conc. to form a lotion content/cream, it is known to greatly inhibit the possible formation of blisters, while relating to burns, when applied immediately and then after every three-hour interval for a period of 4 to 5 days. If you notice any complications during the course of administering this mixture, consult your doctor immediately.

It should be administered topically on the skin or areas of the body where a burn is known to have occurred.

As always mentioned, please ensure you seek the counsel of a qualified health practitioner before administering this recommendation to yourself or anybody else. This is because, just as all humans are made different, that is how our body reacts to things differently.

✤ <u>CRYOPROTECTANT DIMETHYL SULPHOXIDE.</u>

Simply put, a cryoprotectant is a chemical substance that inhibits, avoids possible damage, and halts the freezing of cells and tissues. DMSO is a very good cryoprotectant agent.

DMSO as a cryoprotectant is often used in the prevention of both intracellular and intercellular crystals which are in cells when the freezing process begins. Recent studies have shown that these crystals result in the demise of the cells which in turn will affect possible transplant.

DMSO has also been used in this context as a preservative, in the preservation of cord blood cells, derived from the umbilical cords from childbirth.

In return, these cord blood cells are used in the treatment of many possible medical illnesses, especially in babies. Some of them are;

- ⧗ In treating cerebral palsy.
- ⧗ Traumatic brain injuries/disorder.
- ⧗ Childhood leukemia.

Without a cryoprotectant which DMSO is, these blood cells cannot survive the freezing process. And thereby making them readily available for fast and effective transplant when the medical need arises.

⤷ DMSO FOR THE TREATMENT OF FACIAL ACNE.

Acne is a defective skin condition, that is commonly prevalent in adolescents, and sometimes adults. It normally comes with some pimples, and blemishes which are due to inflammations in the sebaceous glands. Bacterial is a major cause of this skin condition and the various types of acne are; Rosacea, Blackheads, Cystic, and Vulgaris.

The dimethyl sulphoxide is known to be a hindrance to the development/growth of bacteria.

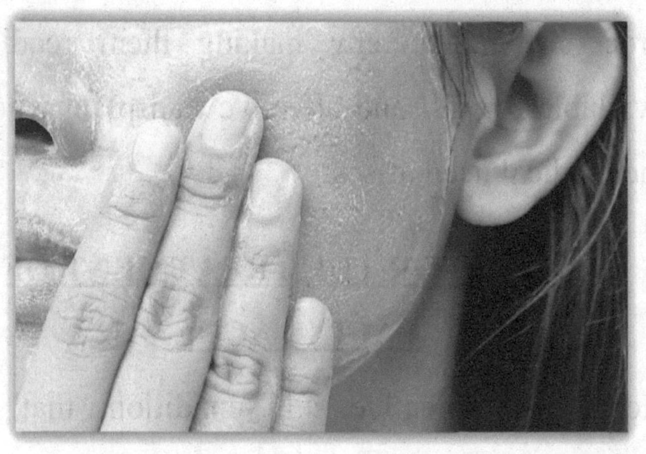

Apply some DMSO with a mixture of aloe-vera in a percentage ratio of 65%:35%. Apply the same topically on the affected area of the body for at least twice daily, for about 14days (you can stop its application, if you notice a good progress with your treatment).

✧ <u>HOW DMSO RELATES TO CELL-BIOLOGY AND THE VITRO-FERTILIZATION PROCESS.</u>

Dimethyl sulfoxide (DMSO) has been known to be a cryoprotectant and is used very extensively in cell-biology. It has good penetrating and displacement properties.

Apart from other usefulness of DMSO, it is also used in laboratories in water-hydrogen bonding-related experiments (which enable it to reduce icing and subsequently eliminate the tendency of cell death).

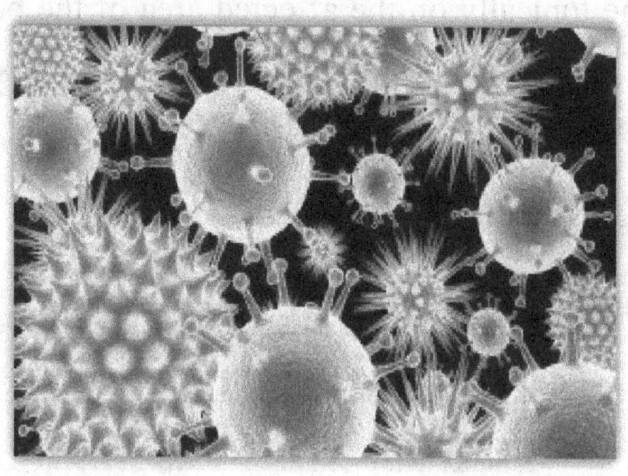

In in-vitro fertilization (IVF), the process of vitrification is achieved when more concentrated portions of cryoprotectants (15% DMSO with 15% ethylene glycol) are used to mitigate the formation of ice in cells and their solutions.

↬ <u>AMYLOIDOSIS.</u>

This is a disease that is grouped as a heterogeneous ailment of inflammatory, chronic underlying infectious symptom(s) related to diseases like rheumatoid arthritis, tuberculosis, and others.

Amyloidosis illnesses are not too easy to diagnose, because their symptoms could be closely related to that of other ailments., particularly in its early stage.

When left unattended, Amyloidosis can have a serious adverse effect on the body's internal organs, both in a systemic or localized way.

Chemotherapy and steroid therapy for this ailment have been the trend before scientists discovered the efficacy of DMSO in the treatment of the disease.

According to research, applying the DMSO liquid topically on the area of amyloidosis in a concentration of 50% mixed with distilled water

of50%, daily for a 3-month cycle.

CHAPTER 4.

ALZHEMER'S, ARTHRITIS, HERPES, SHINGLES, ATHLETIC INHURIES, NERVE PAIN, BRIAN AND DEMENTIA DISEASES.

⇨ ALZHEMER'S

This is a notorious disease that is closely related to the functioning of the brain. If not quickly checked, could lead to the degeneration and death of the brain cells. From research, it has been confirmed that Alzheimer's disease is the most common cause of dementia ailment of the brain.

This disease is mostly associated with persons of old age. A person suffering from dementia experiences a worsening effect when he/she gets older, and sometimes it even gets worse that such persons may even lose the ability to carry out their everyday routine without any help.

As old age sets in, the blood and amyloid circulation diminishes due to a lack of adequate oxygen around the brain area.

⇘ **ARTHRITIS.**

Arthritis is one of the major grounds/causes of rendering persons immobile. Arthritis effects could be minor or severe, depending on the state of the ailment.

Unlike dimethyl sulphoxide which has an aftermath taste, MSM (a chemical substance derived from DMSO) doesn't have such negative side effects. Reports from medical practitioners and patients have revealed that

DMSO application is one of the best ways of treating arthritis ailments.

One of the reasons that gave rise to this conclusion is that dimethyl sulphoxide reduces the pain and possible muscular cramps that are normally felt around the joint areas where arthritis is suspected. Another reason is that the MSM helps to secure, provide, and transport the needed biologically available sulfur to the damaged ligaments of the joint area.

In treating arthritis, DMSO is administered either topically or orally with a concentration ratio of (50%:50%) water to DMSO. For topical application, administer your DMSO.

Also, in treating osteoarthritis, apply topically a 25% DMSO gel on the exact knee or joint locations thrice daily, for a period of 21 days. Do consult your doctor for advice before you use it.

➷ <u>**HERPES AND SHINGLES.**</u>

Shingles also known as Herpes is a disease condition from the family of Genus Varicellovirus. When treated rightly, it will get cleared from the body in less than 21 days. It is best it is treated before it gets to affect the eyes, particularly when the face has been infected, this could lead to blindness.

DMSO sprays (a combination of various anti-inflammatory and antiviral medicines), or solutions of 60% DMSO with 40% water could be applied twice daily on the surface of the body where the shingles are. In the event that you feel pain as a result of the DMSO concentration, you may dilute it more with water.

Also, you can apply about 10% of idoxuridine in a 60% DMSO solution and apply topically on the skin areas where the herpes is present about 3 to 4 times daily. Normally, the positive relief is felt within one week of application.

In treating shingles ailment, topical application is recommended on the spot or in areas where it is noticed. With a concentration of 70% DMSO and 30% idoxuridine, to be applied every 4 to 5 hours for a period of 72 to 96 hours.
Please note that as per standard health-related practice, you should consult a medical health expert for guidance before use.

✥ NERVE PAIN.

The human body is made of a network of bodily nerves. The FDA approved DMSO as a prescription medicine for pain. In treating nerve-related pain, a topical administration should be carried out 4 to 5 times every 24 hours around the most sensitive part of the body where the pain is felt, while gently rubbing the surface.

✍ <u>**ATHLETIC INJURIES.**</u>

As an athlete involved in any track-field event/sports (gymnastics, judo, football, wrestling, swimming, sprint, and so many others), it is very rare for you to be free from occasional athletic-related injuries and abrasions like dislocations, sprains, broken bones, and cuts.

In treating with DMSO, it is recommended that a conc. of between 65 to 70 percent and cortisone or peppermint oil of 25 to 30 percent, should be practically used in the rehabilitation process of these sports-related injuries.

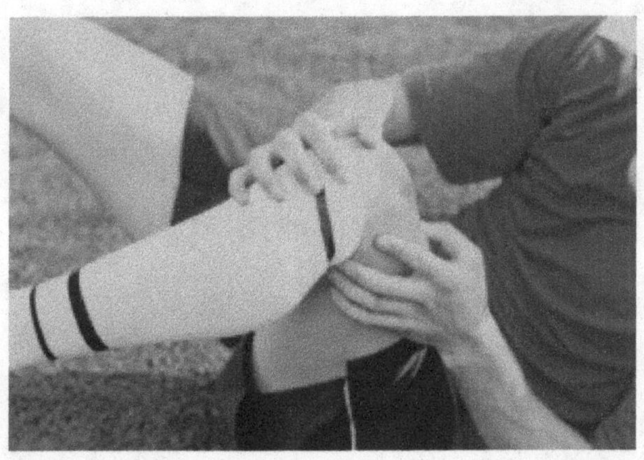

Here, DMSO is advised to be applied topically on the area of pain. However, in some other cases, it is done by spraying. Apply the concentration at every 2hrs interval for the next 8hrs, counting from when the incident occurred.

✎ **<u>BRAIN INJURIES.</u>**

Here, we will be discussing the injuries that may result in brain damage (which may include lack of

oxygen supply, nerve injury, and a reduction in the flow of blood). Some of these wounds/injuries are;

- ⧖ Industrial or vehicular accidents.
- ⧖ Falls.
- ⧖ Trauma.

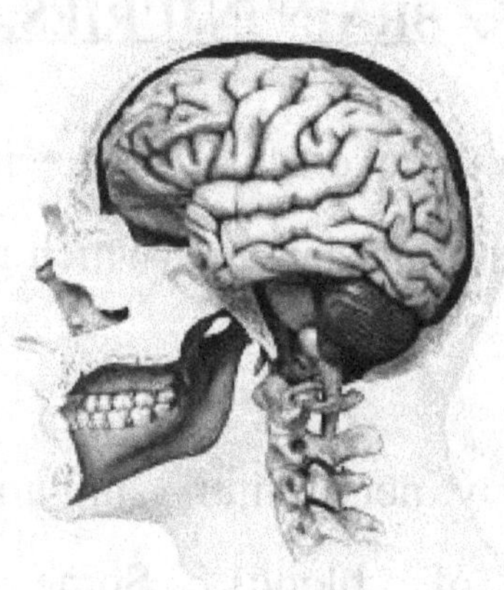

Researchers have found out that the dimethyl sulfoxide is a good chemical compound that is very effective in the treatment of brain-related injuries.

Administering DMSO of 40% concentration to a patient of 40kg weight (in a proportional ratio of 1g to 1kg of the patient). This treatment should be swift to avoid total damage to the brain, which in some cases could lead to death.

However, consult a certified medical expert for advice before you administer this drug.

When the brain has a fatal injury, due to the fragile nature of its tissues, it is deprived of adequate oxygen. The dimethyl sulfoxide is a major/unique agent for the treatment of some of these brain injuries, as a result of some of its unique physical and chemical properties.

In administering the drug to a patient with brain injury, it is done intravenously (through a drip), under the supervision of a medical expert. For a very severe case of brain injuries, one kilogram of a person's body weight to 5grms of DMSO, and the patient should be observed for any possible side effect(s), for the first 24hrs.

After the first day, the dosage should be reduced to 2grms of DMSO per one kg of the patient's body weight.

CHAPTER 5.

BURNS, CANCER, CARPAL TUNNEL SYNDROME, AND CIRRHOSIS OF THE LIVER.

Any injury that causes bodily damage to the skin or its tissue to have primarily been as a result of heat, is called a burn. Now, this heat could be as a result of exposure to the body sun, radiation, fire, electrical or chemical substances, and others.

Burns could be major or minor. Some examples of   minor burns could be sun-burns, scalds, little blister burns, and other burns that can be treated with the help of a first-aid. Examples of major burns could be deep and wide cut, which will need the immediate attention of a specialized burns-expert, as this could take a long time to heal.

According to scientists, research was conducted in the late nineteenth century while comparing the efficacy of the DMSO drug on burns treatment, against other conventional drugs for burns treatment like Monomycin and Nitrofurazone, and it was found out that DMSO showed more efficacy in healing than those other drugs which it was compared to.

It was noticed that DMSO dissolves faster in the body, and helps to prevent the formation of scar tissues in the body.

✎ <u>CANCER AND CANCEROUS GROWTH.</u>

Over forty years ago, a group of researchers due to the proven chemical properties of DMSO, administered the drug to a cancer patient, along with amino acids, and cyclophosphamide, and they noticed a great improvement. The chemotherapeutic properties of the dimethyl sulfoxide drug have further proven the efficacy of this wonder drug.

Testimonies attesting to this fact have been published, both in the online and print media worldwide. DMSO is known to improve the supply of blood through a dilating process (particularly of the smaller blood vessels in the lower limb region).

DMSO is a detoxification agent, a removal of free radicals, and when administered with other chemical compounds as stated above to form a drug, it shows its eliminating powers on cancerous cells, as a result of its penetrating and potentiating properties.

To administer this treatment, an 80% DMSO mixed with 10% amino acids, and 10% cyclophosphamide, should be administered topically with the strict supervision of a qualified medical practitioner.

Get this done in an interval of between 5hrs to 8hrs, for a period of two weeks.

✎ **<u>CARPAL TUNNEL SYNDROME.</u>**

Carpal Tunnel Syndrome (CTS), is an occurring strain injury that happens normally in the knee, elbow, and ankle regions of the body.

In the body physiology, the median nerve located around the wrist of the hand which enables physical feelings, movement, and sense of touch, experiences compression. This results in some severe pain, hand and arm tingling, and weakness of bodily muscles particularly the hands and fingers. The nerve can get damaged permanently if the compression prolongs, which in some could lead to paralysis of the hand or arm wrist region.

Researchers discovered that a chemical compound which is known as Methylsulfonylmethane (MSM), which is derived from the human body and some foods, when used with Dimethylsulphoxide (DMSO), was very helpful in successful medical surgery.

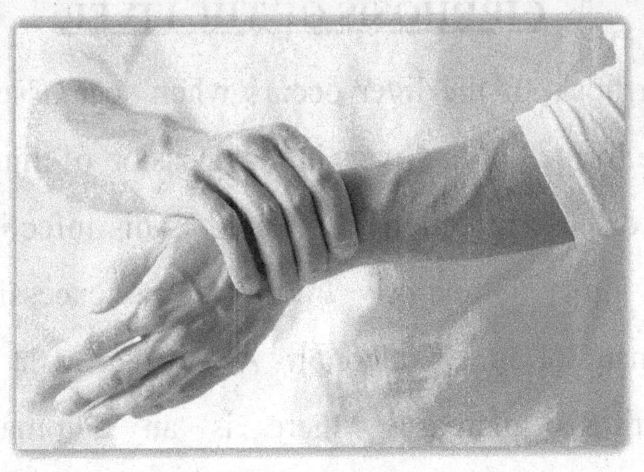

The dimethylsulphoxide which is a very good and effective anti-inflammatory agent, helps to prevent the possibility of any inflammation on the wrist, which could have caused the compression of the median nerve.

Apply DMSO from the finger region, through to the elbow area 2 to 4 times a day. Topically administer the drug to the patient for a period of three weeks.

↳ **CIRRHOSIS OF THE LIVER.**

Cirrhosis of the liver occurs when scar tissues are formed in the liver, in the occasion of injury or disease infection to the liver. This infection or injury is majorly traced to the excessive consumption of alcohol. As the growth of cirrhosis increases, there is an automatic increase in the formation of the scar tissue. This could ultimately lead to the death of the human when not carefully and quickly attended to.

To treat, administer one teaspoon of the mixture from a concentration of 50% DMSO and 50% Aloe-vera to a cirrhosis sufferer. Apply orally twice a day for half a year, or until you get the best expected result. This should be done under the strict supervision of a certified medical expert.

CHAPTER 6.

DIABETES, DIGESTIVE, EAR & EYE INFECTIONS PROBLEMS.

✍ DIABETES.

Diabetes is a disease condition that results, when the organ in the body called the pancreas, finds it difficult to produce the right amount of insulin that is needed by the body, or in another case when the body cannot effectively utilize the amount of insulin as produced by the pancreas.

Simply put, insulin is a hormone in the body that helps to regulate the amount of glucose, secreted or produced by the body.

According to the World Health Organization (WHO), between the years 2000 and 2009, the world recorded a 3% increase in the death rate from cases of diabetes, and 13% of this rate came from lower-income countries.

There are basically three types of diabetes viz-a-viz;

- **<u>Type 1 Diabetes:</u>** This is characterized by a situation of deficient insulin secretion or production by the pancreas.
- **<u>Type 2 Diabetes:</u>** This stops the human body from utilizing the insulin produced by the pancreas properly, which could lead to damage of the blood vessels, if not treated urgently.
- **<u>Gestational Diabetes:</u>** This occurs mostly in pregnant women. Gestational

diabetes results when the blood sugar level is above normal, but below the diagnostic tendency for a diabetic situation.

To treat, apply DMSO topically on part of the body (as closely monitored and advised by a certified health expert), three times daily.

In other cases, you may choose to take a teaspoon of DMSO mixed with some juice for better taste, at a ratio of 50% DMSO to 50% juice, once every day for about half a year.
You should consult your healthcare provider for adequate guidance before you embark on this treatment.

✍ <u>**DIGESTIVE PROBLEMS.**</u>

DMSO in the treatment of digestive-related Problems. Indigestion could be a very disturbing and uncomfortable health condition when prolonged. It could lead to excessive flatulence.

Research has shown that dimethylsulphoxide (DMSO) could reduce the negative side effects of indigestion in no small way, particularly when it is mixed with Aloe-vera.

Get to mix a half teaspoon of DMSO in two ounces of pure Aloe-vera juice, shake thoroughly for a proper blend, and drink twice daily, preferably after you have had your breakfast, and dinner as well, for a period of 21 days.

⤼ **EAR INFECTIONS.**

Viruses to which the ears are exposed, often time cause ear infection(s). These infections if left unattended for a long period, could lead to chronic hearing impairment, which in most cases are treated with surgical operations. These surgeries are in most cases expensive and painful to the patient.

But with the use of the Dimethylsulphoxide (DMSO) which according to research, when it is mixed with an anesthetic drug, helps to reduce the pain and resultant negative side effects of the surgical operation.

Further studies have shown that the DMSO can be successfully used to treat some ear infections when it is combined with some antibiotics without any surgical operations on the ear. An ear-dropper is usually the instrument used in facilitating this treatment.

With the proper supervision of a medical expert, get a 50% DMSO solution, use an ear-dropper, and apply 1 to 2 drops onto the ear that is infected.

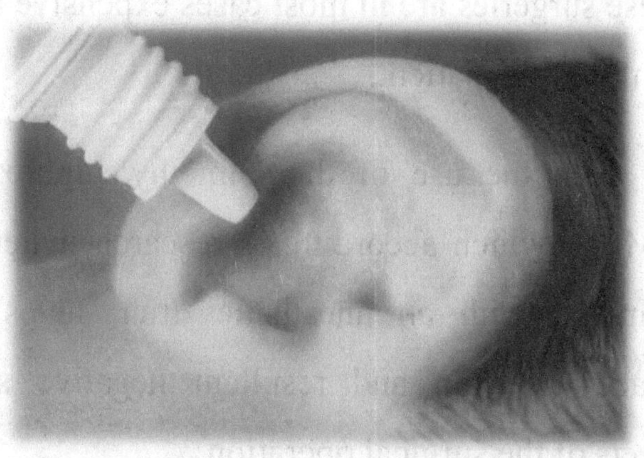

Researchers have discovered that when an 80% DMSO and Aloe-vera was administered dermally/topically to the ear region, neck, and head area of the patient, this gives a whole lot of relief, particularly to children.

↳ __EYE DISEASES.__

The dimethylsulphoxide (DMSO) has in no small way aided the treatment of eye-related diseases that hitherto affect the eyes and its component parts harmfully. Some of these eye ailments include glaucoma, eye cataracts, retina deterioration, and others, which could result in permanent blindness if left unattended.

This amazing DMSO medication can be applied topically to treat conditions like cataracts and glaucoma. Research indicates that other doctors have also experienced success by injecting one drop of a sterile physiologic or saline solution containing 25 mg of DMSO and 2cc of Superoxide Dismutase (SOD) into each eyeball once or twice a day for ten days. This method is effective for curing cataracts, glaucoma, and other vision-related issues as well as for treating pain in the eyes.

CHAPTER 7.

<u>FIBROMYALAGIA, FUNGUS, HAIR-SCALP, AND HEADACHES.</u>

This is an ailment that causes very serious pain to the muscular parts of the body like the back, shoulders, arms, necks, and legs as well. This could lead to a worrisome, overbearing tiredness, and possible malfunctioning of the body's nervous system, which includes the ligaments, and tendons.

This disease can happen to both genders and the chances of having the disease increase with time. The disease is not an easy one to diagnose due to the similarities in symptoms with other diseases.

According to medical research, the element sulfur serves as a very good reliever for sufferers of pains within the body parts discussed above, particularly bones and muscles by detoxification and collagen production.

Methylsulfonylmethane (MSM) is derived from a sulphuric compound closely affiliated with DMSO (dimethyl sulphoxide). To administer this drug to the sufferer of fibromyalgia, apply topically to the areas of the body where you experience chronic pain.

A patient was diagnosed with fibromyalgia ailment and she was administered some painkillers which had some adverse side effects on her. After some time, she was placed on treatment with the dimethylsulphoxide compound.

She was administered this drug intravenously at first, through drip. This drip procedure continued for about eight to ten weeks, for about 3hours per session, and a great improvement was seen.

She also combined a DMSO/JUICE ratio of (50%:50%), for another 10 weeks after the intravenous administration, and positive changes were seen over the years on her.

✎ __DMSO AS AN ANTI-FUNGAE AGENT.__

Over the years, the chemical compound DMSO has been discovered to be a very valuable and effective medicine, whether when it is used alone in the treatment of diseases, or when it is used in a combined state.

As an antifungal agent, DMSO can also be combined with iodine; a griseofulvin antibiotic agent, to form a concentrated solution.

DMSO can be used to treat a fungus-infested skin, but you will to consult your health service provider, for possible guidance on how you can go about it.

✎ __HAIR AND SCALP PROBLEMS.__

One of the best properties of dimethylsulphoxide (DSMO), is the fact that it has the ability to trigger/induce the growth of hair particularly in areas/region of the body where there are stunted growth or lack of hair.

Cancer patients and individuals who as a result of their chemotherapy have had loss of hair, have experienced speedy hair regrowth when they used the DMSO concentrated solution. This rapid regrowth, according to scientific research develops in a period of six months.

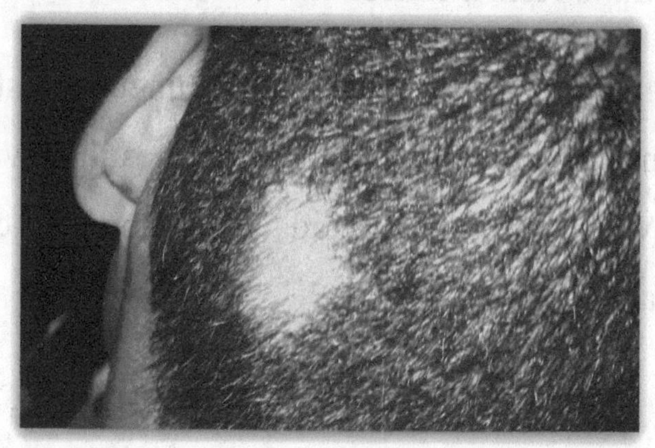

Administer DMSO of 50% cc. to the affected region on your skin in the area where the scalp is affected. Do this every day (twice a day for a period of 12 weeks to 24 weeks).

☞ __HEADACHES.__

Headaches are generally discomforting. They are caused by excessive muscular contractions around the neck region, emotional stress, and shoulders as well as changes in the blood vessels that lead to the head.

There are different types of headaches; migraines could even affect a section of the head (the eyes, nose, tension headaches, sinus headaches, cluster, chronic daily headaches, e.t.c and these could be very frustrating.

Scientists made some good research about the effectiveness of DMSO on headaches and it was observed that the level of therapeutic healing the patient or individual felt was very tremendous.

To treat, get a blend of DMSO of 75% cc and distilled water of 25% cc. Administer the solution topically on the back of the neck area or the area of the pain where such headache pain is been experienced. Some persons may want to use cotton wool to apply. Relieve can be noticed within 24hrs of this application.

CHAPTER 8.

INTERSTITIAL CYSTITIS, LUPUS, STROKE, SPINAL CORD, TOOTH & GUM DISEASES.

✎ **<u>INTERSTITIAL CYSTITIS.</u>**

Interstitial Cystitis (IC) is a health condition that is often time erroneously taken to be a urinary tract infection (UTI), but in actual reality, it isn't. This disease condition is known to affect more women (particularly women of age-bearing age), than it affects men.

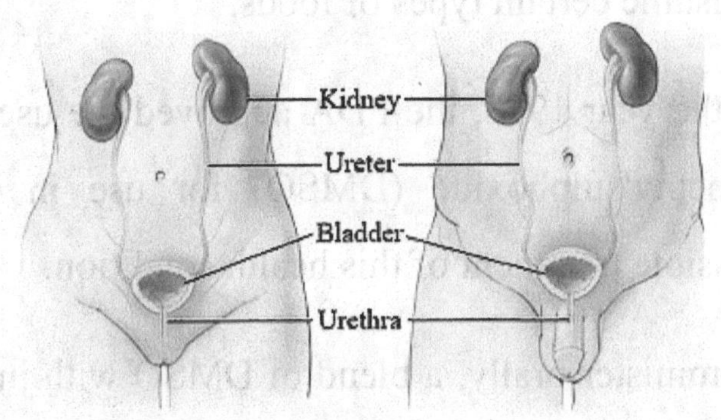

Interstitial Cystitis is a chronic inflamed bladder wall disorder, that often time than not, leads to bladder hardening and makes it

difficult for urine to be held in the bladder, thereby leading to frequent urination.

To this day, it is quite difficult for medical researchers to know what the possible causes of this disease condition could be, although some patients of this disease are said to have noticed increased worsening conditions when they consume certain types of foods.

In the year 1978, the FDA approved the use of dimethylsulphoxide (DMSO) for use in the possible treatment of this health condition.

Administer orally, a blend of DMSO with juice or water in a 50:50 ratio. Take a teaspoon of such blend twice a day for 21 days. But consult your doctor for guidance before you administer such, just in case you have some underlying health conditions.

✥ <u>LUPUS.</u>

Lupus is an inflammatory health condition that is closely with the connective tissues that affect the bladder, skin, and other internal organs in the body (such as the kidney).

Some of the symptoms of this disease include frequent fever, tiredness, scaly and dried skin, and pains in the joint area.

Treatment of this disease with the dimethylsulphoxide (DMSO), has demonstrated a great level of improvement in sufferers of this disease condition. Apply DMSO solution dermally on the joint areas where you experience such pain, under the close supervision of your medical advisor, till you get the desired result which you wish for.

⤷ <u>STROKE, AND SPINAL CORD INJURIES.</u>

Stroke is a disease condition that occurs in a situation when the blood that normally flows to the brain is unexpectedly blocked due to vessel damage, and this is known as ischemic stroke. It can also occur when there is bleeding in the brain.

If not tackled or treated on time, it can lead to a lethal consequence. So, it should be best handled at the minimal level, when it just started. Dimethylsulphoxide (DMSO) has been known for decades to provide a good remedy for this disease.

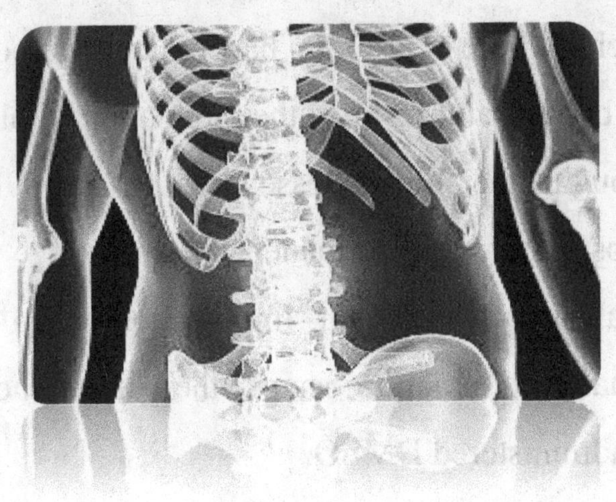

DMSO has a characteristic penetrating ability of being able to move beyond the blood-brain barrier protector. With this, the dimethylsulphoxide enables and helps other blood vessels to take up the responsibility of transporting blood to the brain, in the absence of the damaged blood vessels.

When administered intravenously, particularly within the first few hours of the case being reported, the DMSO permeates the body and reaches the blood-brain barrier area, removes the barrier, and restores the circulation of blood through other blood vessels to the brain. This helps to forestall permanent brain damage and paralysis of the patient. Immediately when this spinal cord situation occurs, the patient should be administered DMSO.

✎ <u>TOOTH AND GUM DISEASE.</u>

When the refined sugar/sweetened food eaten remains in the teeth for a long period of time without removal, bacteria grow.

And these bacteria nourish themselves on the gum walls of the teeth, within the mouth. This mouth times can cause bleeding and sometimes could spread to other membranes in the mouth, which could lead to the removal of tooth or teeth.

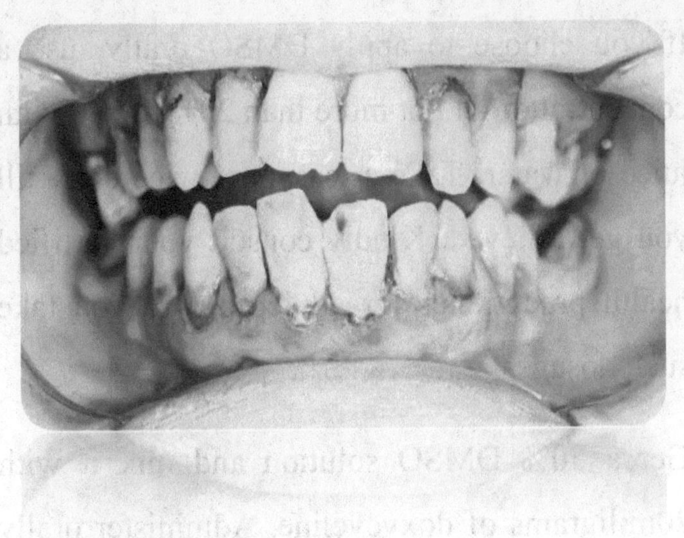

Apply topically a DMSO concentration of 80 to 90% for the areas of the body that aren't sensitive as earlier mentioned. And a lower concentration of about 50 to 60% and the other percentage ratio of aloe-vera, can be used in those other bodily regions/parts. Administer the blend twice to thrice in a day, until the recovery you desire is realized.

If you choose to apply DMSO orally, use a concentration of not more than 20% mixed with juice or water. Take a teaspoon twice daily till you get relieved. Kindly consult your certified health practitioner for advice before you take such dosages.

Get a 50% DMSO solution and mix it with 20miligrams of doxycycline. Administer orally into the mouth and rinse your mouth with it, while guiding the solution to the part of the mouth where the pain is felt.

Get your mouth rinsed thoroughly with a small portion of this solution for about 3 minutes and spew it out from your mouth. Desist from swallowing the concentration.

However, this should be done under the supervision of your healthcare provider for effective management.

Toothache or decay occurs when molded bacteria are formed in the tooth or gums of the mouth. Research has it that excessive consumption of processed/refined sweetened foods, over a long period, with adequate teeth brushing, could lead to toothache/decay.

Periodontal tooth disease is a major factor that causes tooth loss in the elderly. Brushing your teeth regularly could help in no small way to reduce bacterial growth on the tooth.

CHAPTER 9.

STORAGE & INDUSTRIAL USE OF DMSO.

✏ DMSO As A Cleaning Agent & Processing Agent:

Industrially, DMSO due to its solubility characteristic is a good non-toxic cleaning solvent, particularly in the removal of tough stains and organic chemical substances from machines, production lines/equipment, and as a paint stripper from surfaces.

Research shows that it is also good in polymer membrane and synthetic fibers production, where it can be used as a processing solvent.

↳ **DMSO As A Radiation Protective Agent.**

Radiation and radioactive elements are known to produce dangerous free-radicals which are very harmful to man's health, and uncontrolled exposure to these radiations either directly or indirectly could lead to some cancerous growth, avoidable birth defects in infants, and increased cases of ill-health.

For decades, dimethylsulphoxide (DMSO) has been used as a protective agent against radioactive-related elements.

Administering DMSO in this condition could be done via the three modes of application (orally, topically, or intravenously), depending on the one prescribed for you by your doctor.

For radiations or exposures that are named chronic, more concentrated dosages of DMSO are recommended (excluding the face and other vital/sensitive parts of the body).

HOW TO STORE DMSO?

DMSO is a universal solvent. Research has shown that when you want to apply DMSO on an open/exposed injury or in areas of the body that are sensitive as explained earlier in one of the paragraphs above, it is best you use a lower/weaker concentration of DMSO.

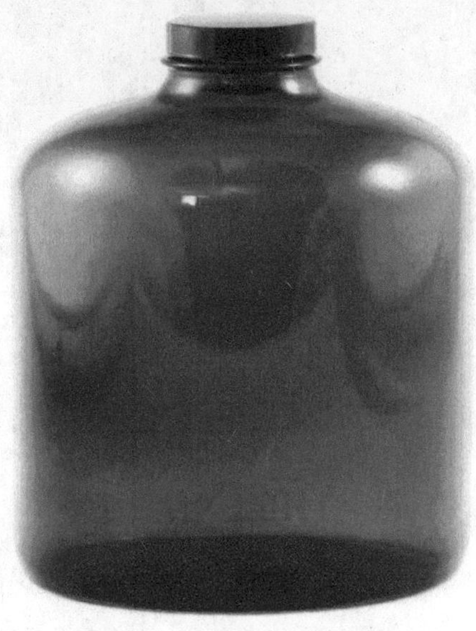

Don't forget that water, juice, and Aloe-vera are still one of the best mixing companions with DMSO.

DMSO is better stored or preserved in glass or polyethylene plastic containers such as HDPE, PTFE, PP, and PETE.

DMSO should be stored in a dry cool place, free from fire, and kept out of the reach of children.

THE END.